MEMOIRS
of
A Kenyan Yogi

MEMOIRS
of
A Kenyan Yogi

by
Cheloti Kennedy Wamalwa Kundu

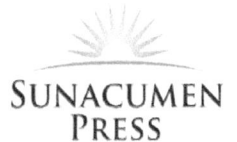

SUNACUMEN
PRESS

Copyright 2020 © Cheloti Kennedy Wamalwa Kundu
All rights reserved.

No part of this publication may be reproduced, stored in a retrieval system, or transmitted, in any form or by any means, without the prior permission in writing of Cheloti Kennedy Wamalwa Kundu, or as expressly permitted by law.

Cover photos by Evans Ombisa
Cover and interior design by Sunacumen Press
Palm Springs, CA
www.sunacumenpress.com

ISBN 13: 978-0-9995612-9-4

Printed in U.S.A.

Contents

Introduction   9
How a somersault bought me a ticket to art   11
How yoga found me   21
The impact of yoga on my life   25
My interpretation of yoga   33
Yoga with African traditions and culture   37
My early days in yoga   41
Makutano junction   47
The shepherds   57
My lie   61
The system does not define you   67
Trust the process   79
The modern warrior   83
Disrupting the soil   87
Highlights   91
Relationships   95
Packing   99
The konga   103
When life shakes you   105
Acknowledgments   111

Dedication

To all the women in my life

Introduction

My name is Cheloti, and I am a proud father of two beautiful girls, Chilande and Wanjiku, who are now eight and six years old. I am a certified Level 3 yoga instructor from the Africa Yoga Project and Baptiste Yoga Institute and the first to be a certified acro-yoga international teacher in Africa. I have been a professional acrobat for the past fifteen years, and these days, I like to call myself a "retired general." I have since transitioned from active acrobatic performance to teaching yoga and acro yoga. My greatest joy is seeing people work together and supporting each other to create abundance in everything around them. This is where my love for the community is founded. My dream is to build a global yoga and acro yoga village and bring meaning to the phrase, "one world, one people, one love."

My purpose is to hold the mantle of equality and simplicity, to unveil hidden opportunities through self-realization and discovery. To create a platform where communal support is available to access the greatest potential in all. I teach through my and other people's experiences. These different experiences give a more varied and broader approach to our way of thinking and way of being. This is done in the hopes of challenging us into nonconformity and pushing us to learn to seek answers from within.

How a Somersault Bought Me a Ticket to Art

My life as a performing artist was not planned, but rather born of necessity. Four months before I was hired by the Safari Park Hotel as a dancer, I was retrenched from my first job as an electrician at Simmers Restaurant in the city center of Nairobi. Those four months were the most difficult I have ever spent in my life. Paying rent became an insurmountable task, and many nights went by without food on my table. I lost my close circle of friends and had to make new ones to survive. I survived by doing odd jobs and favors that I would not have done if I had a choice. I had to do many odd jobs just to get enough money for food—which was not a lot back then—from unblocking old sewage lines to clearing road drainage systems, a job that was actually meant for city council workers. Hired as cheap labor for the price of a meal or less, I was paid whatever my employer deemed fit, but never above a dollar. Nevertheless, it was a penny I would not have had and one that secured a warm meal at a roadside cafe. These penny jobs were rare, and you were lucky to get one.

After three and a half months of playing hide and seek with

my landlord, I was served with a two-week eviction notice. Staying in a single room in Umoja Estate in Eastlands with a communal bathroom, toilet and a utensils basin was no longer possible.

Eastlando, as it is known among the locals, is made up of a mixture of both middle-lower-class and lower-class citizens. Most of the middle-lower class citizens are former government employees who worked for the municipal council and railway transportation company before it was taken over by the private sector. Over time the area has slowly transformed into a lower-class habitat. A big percentage of the population is jobless, which encourages a lot of theft and muggings from as early as 6:30 pm on. When the sun went down, an array of illegal drugs hit the streets. This trade is one of the many activities that went on in the dark hours.

I am not entirely sure how I stayed away from the gangs, but I think it was because I was too much of a coward. I couldn't picture myself hurting someone else to get by. I witnessed most of the "night action" many times over. I stayed out late on most occasions, way past midnight, before retreating to my small dingy room. These "night actions" scared me, but the thought of no shelter terrified me more. Life can be interesting.

In the early days of losing my job, I approached friends and relatives easily. They understood my situation, and they sympathized with me. However, after two weeks, they got tired of seeing me, and many of them simply chose to avoid me. That is when you know things have changed around you. After that, I also started hiding from them because of the things I had to do to survive.

"I wish I had somebody who cared," I thought. I craved the warmth of a family, community, and people who could listen to my cries. I wished I had somewhere to run to, but my family was struggling just as much as I was. It seemed like everybody I knew was struggling, and the expression "die like a man" gave shape and meaning to what was happening to me at the time.

At the Safari Park Hotel, where I had gone to drop off one of my many application letters, I discovered that a dance audition was ongoing, and I asked if I could try my luck as well. I needed a job, anything at all that could put a roof over my head and food on my table. The day before, the only food that I ate was from "gate-crashing" a wedding. In Kenya, weddings are an open invitation. If you ever happen to have yours in Kenya, know that you have invited everyone, unless you have security at the gate to keep unwanted guests away.

So, when I was given a chance to try, I gave it my all. At the audition, the supervisor was tired of seeing the same dance from everybody and asked me to do something different, a somersault or breakdance move. The last time I had tried something like this was when I was about ten years old. But you see, I had nothing to lose. I had no meals to go back to and was looking at an eviction in two weeks. I had hit rock bottom. I was so desperate I could have done anything. Yes, I was scared beyond words, but that is not what came out of my mouth. I told the supervisor that I could do it. I psyched myself up mentally, told people to move out of my way, and I went for it. Well, I did turn in the air except my head was just a few inches off the ground. I barely landed on my feet as part of my bum connected to the floor.

Everyone gasped, shocked that I would even dare to pull such a stunt with no skill at all. The supervisor asked if I was okay. You would think he would have mercy and not ask me to repeat it, right? Wrong! That is exactly what he asked me to do. He asked if I could do it again.

A little hesitant, I said I could. In that split second we locked eyes, and whatever he saw in my eyes must have scared him. As I moved backward to create even more space, he asked me to stop for a moment.

"Are sure you can do this?" he asked. I heard, "Go home if you can't do it."

I shouted, "No, I mean yes, yes I can." Although I said this aloud, maybe too loud, the answer was more to myself than to him. With all the courage and bravery that I could summon, I went for it again.

I ran diagonally across the room, and in the middle of the room leaped up into the air, somersaulted, and landed on my feet. Everybody stood up clapping and cheering, some screaming out loud, "Yay!"

I stood there. I couldn't move. It was as if I was glued to the floor. I heard a voice over the claps. "Well, young man, you just proved how much you want this job. You have your chance, for now. Two weeks is all you have to catch up with the rest of the team. If you don't, unfortunately, even with your devil determination, I will not keep you." With that, the supervisor left the room. I wiped my tears, hoping to conceal my emotions. Too late; everybody seemed to know exactly what was going on.

This is how I began my artistic life. I literally somersaulted into the world of art. Les Brown, a motivational speaker, shares in one of his talks, "You gotta be hungry if you want to do anything worthwhile in life." Hungry people don't stop until they get it because they are highly motivated. You've got to be willing to stay through the pain and focus only on what you want and where your inspiration comes from. Find your "why," and that will give you the motivation to push forward. Had I focused instead on the humiliation after the first somersault, I would not have tried the second time.

After getting confirmation that I had gotten the job, I asked a friend for a financial boost so that I could move closer to my new job, and out of the house in Umoja. I moved out in a week's time to a small house in Githurai 44 on a monthly allowance of 1,800 shillings from my new dancing job, an equivalent of eighteen dollars a month. Githurai 44 is along Thika highway and past Safari Park Hotel where I was now working. I paid twelve dollars for rent and six dollars for a month's worth of food. My elder brother was also rotting upcountry in the village, so I asked him to come to stay with me. This house was tinier than the previous one in Umoja, but, guess what: life goes on.

Six months down the line, I was training in acrobatics with a few of my friends. An additional six months saw us transition fully from dancing into acrobatic training. This is when life became interesting again. Three of us had just quit our jobs to train as acrobats.

See, there comes a time in life when you have to take the plunge, this was that time for us. Like Anais Nin said, "And the day came when the risk it took to remain tight in the bud was more painful than the risk it took to blossom."

Don't get me wrong, Safari Park was a good place to be and work. We just did not see a future in dancing there, and in Kenya in general at the time, so we chose to try our luck in acrobatics. It is not like we were going to college or a school for acrobatics. We went out training on our own, following and asking for guidance from other acrobatic groups that we knew around us. We went in without holding back. We trained like there was no tomorrow. We had so much confidence and belief in ourselves. We were so sure that we would make it through to be among the recognized groups of acrobats, despite the fact that we started training late in life. We were all over twenty years old, and one of us was thirty-two years old at the time. We relied heavily on our dancing background and hoped this would give us an upper hand in the trade, and it did. Fusing both dance and acrobatics gave us an edge over the others. It also helped that we trained two times a day and for long hours. Our program looked something like this:

5:45-6:30 am: Morning run
8:30-12:00 pm: Morning skill training
12-2:15 pm: Break for "lunch" (rest with no food)
2:15-4:00 pm: Afternoon skill training
Break for home
8 pm-9 pm: Evening strength building, dinner, and bed.

This schedule continued for six months nonstop, fueled by the constant reminder of people on the sidelines telling us that we were too old to make a mark in the field of art. We knew we had no choice but to work hard and prove them wrong. There was no quitting. We worked with our eyes firmly fixed on our goal, which was to get a contract outside the country. With a well-wishers blessing of 30,000 shillings, an equivalent of 300 dollars, we received during the first six months of training, it was possible to concentrate on creating and perfecting our show. After six months of living on a minimal budget, we ran out of cash and had to find work for food, housing and all else that was needed.

As we progressed in our practice, things started becoming really hard for us. One of our group members came back with a letter from the doctor advising him to stop training in acrobatics. We could have quit at this point, but we were too driven to stop. It is then that we realized how art, and specifically acrobatics, was perceived around town. We barely made any money despite our offers to audition or perform without payment for our first show. We encouraged each other to stay strong and believed in the saying, "It gets darker just before dawn." In some venues, we had to settle for a plate of rice and a glass of water and call it a day. But it was much better than nothing, if you ask me.

Later on, as we labored on in our art, we got somewhat better deals where we were paid 2,500 shillings, an equivalent of twenty-five dollars per show. Remember, we were a team of seven men, and 10 percent of our earnings went to the group's upkeep, with the remaining cash divided among ourselves. We each landed with around 300 shillings or three dollars. This disturbed and worried us a lot. If you remember, those of us who started at the Safari Park Hotel got into acrobatics so that we could better our chances of survival. This did not look like an improvement, my friends. We were simply surviving.

History repeats itself, and I found myself reliving my past experience before I went into the art industry. Except for this time, it was better because I had a group of close friends with me. We fought hard battles day after day, knowing at some point our efforts would pay off. We never gave up, always reminding ourselves that one day we would look back and smile with the satisfaction of success running through our souls. Days came and went. One day, I remember I had only twenty shillings in my pocket as we were walking back home from one of our training centers. I was so hungry and tired that I wanted to spend it to buy a donut by the roadside. My friend Job reminded me that it was the only cash we had and we were better off keeping it for supper later that evening. Ten shillings was enough for the two of us to buy mandondo (boiled beans), to eat with ugali, our staple food. The remaining ten shillings was enough for a spliff to bury our problems, or at least numb us enough to get some sleep. The morning would sort itself out, I thought, and life goes on.

The hard work bore fruit. Within the next year, we hit the limelight as a group of upcoming artists. Patience, persistence, and staying focused had finally paid off. We got our first contract outside the country after two years and four months of sweat and tears. We found hope. When you find your passion, do it wholeheartedly. Pay attention to your attitude, it forms part of your drive.

My life as an artist was born out of necessity. I needed a job or something to earn money to buy food and clothing. A place to rest my head when the sun goes down. Four months can seem like years when you don't have money for basic needs. When you have been in such a position in life, mentorship becomes very important. This is why community is so important to me, as we can create and mentor each other from this space. Most people who have made it in life have done so with the help of others who have been through the same or similar situations. We had none of that, and we moved from one hole to the next, or, as one might say, "from the frying pan to the fire."

In our next phase as performers, we made some money. The blueprint from which we operated as people totally dictated our approach. As people who were searching for and struggling to make a living in our previous phase, how do you think we fared? See, when it came to money most of us still operated from the very paradigm we learned when we were young. We knew scarcity, such that we were still looking for money even when we had it or had a way of making it. Wallace D. Wattles writes in his book, *The Science of Getting Rich,* that we are programmed in three primary ways about cash: what we hear when we are young; what we saw when we were young, and what we experienced when we were young.

Some people, because of this blueprint for scarcity, have vowed not to be broke and have devised ways to make money in any way possible. Sometimes, unfortunately, this is done with total disregard for what is the right way of earning or making money. Such people will easily make lots of money and lose it just as fast, and/or not be able to save or do anything tangible with it. If your blueprint led you to believe that good money was unattainable to you or your family, you would then work so hard just to prove them wrong. There is nothing wrong with either way of making money, just that you might think differently if you knew where your motivation was rooted. If you have not tried to understand your blueprint concerning money, there is a chance that you are operating from default; that is, your early childhood belief about money. This, in turn, might be the reason why money is such a complicated issue for you. At least, this is how it was for me.

As a performing artist money was a big issue for me. Looking back, I don't think I was well equipped to handle it. The money came through my hands and left unceremoniously. In a short span of time, when I thought I had it, I lost it. I did not gamble, nor was I a spent-thrift, but somehow, I could hardly hold money down, let alone find a way to grow it. It was as if somebody was stealing from me. But no, I just spent it all. Down in my home village, that would have earned me an appointment with a witch doctor. I was bewitched. "Somebody is behind the disappearance of my money." Money was like fireballs in my hand; I wanted to spend it all fast before I got burned!

Cash was a constant worry. Because of my limiting belief of scarcity, I could not bring myself to go beyond holding money in the bank to investing it. Two months after coming back from abroad, I started worrying about the next few months. What will I eat if I invest this little remaining money? I shied away from any investment ideas because I had limited information about it, and this scared me. I convinced myself this would not work for me or for us as an artistic group that was always on the move. My fear of losing money stopped me from talking to financial advisors. I thought they knew so much that they would con me out of my little cash. As for friends, I thought if they knew how much I had, they would want to borrow the little that I had, or worse, rob me at knife or gunpoint. I was paranoid, no idea was safe.

Now, when I look back, I can't help thinking how much better off I would be if I had been open-minded and knew how to ask for help. However, every lesson has its revelation time, and when it is your time, you will seek out the information you need that will allow you to make the best decisions. Tim Cork says in his book, *G3: The Gift of You, Leadership and Net Giving*: "Simply stated, the money will come if you find your passion. Find what you love and spend your time and focus there."

My advice is to take time to understand what your subconscious thoughts about money are. Make conscious choices about how to go about advancing yourself as a person and positively influencing the people closest to you. Always think of how you can give back. Spend time with the experts and coaches who do this for a living and ask successful people how they got to where they are. Most people will be happy to tell you. If you don't ask, you don't get, and remember it's not just what you ask, but how you ask what you ask for.

How Yoga Found Me

I was re-introduced to yoga through a friend of a friend, an old man of seventy-five years from Bermuda known to me only as Swami. He spent some time with us in Kenya at my friends' place in Nairobi. My friend, Job, and I listened to Swami as he told us about his travels to East Africa in search of the sun. He did sun yoga. It energized him, just as physical exercise will do for you. We thought that was weird and did not understand why he made such a big deal about the sun. But Swami explained to us that every morning as the sun came up, after a little exposure and practice, he would transform from a frail old man into someone full of strength who could walk for miles and never wear out.

I say I was "re-introduced" to yoga because we had come across yoga five years before, as a group, but decided that it was not our thing. At the time we were traveling as performing artists and thought that yoga would make us too flexible and that this would make us more vulnerable to injury. Mostly though, we thought yoga was for women and individualistic people. We played prosecution, judge and jury, case closed. We were so full of ourselves back then—young and ignorant.

There were days we sat and spoke with Swami about the differences between his country and other countries where he had traveled. We discussed the challenges that we faced as young men in Nairobi and Swami told us that, given our background in art and what we had gone through in life, we would discover our strengths, and learn to convert our passion into profits through yoga.

He did not stop there, he practically dragged us to a yoga studio. The studio was in Parklands, called the Africa Yoga Project. He introduced us to the administration and told them our story. As we saw Swami off, he made us promise to practice yoga for at least three months. I was now curious enough about yoga that I wanted to see what options it could provide me.

Shortly after, a yoga teacher named Evans came to our community training hall. We decided that we would enroll in two classes a week for beginners. Over the next month of classes, we got better and better as a team. I enjoyed learning and practicing, and Evans was an amazing teacher and soon a good friend.

For a long time, I had thought yoga to be "girly," but I was so wrong. Coming from a background of intense physical practice you would have thought that yoga would be easy for me. Ha! Yoga kicked my butt. I would sweat and shake like a leaf each time I did a downward-facing dog. It was amazing to discover so much about my body, and to my biggest surprise, I found myself looking at transitioning into teaching yoga. I just didn't know how to go about it at the time. Little did I know that yoga would become my passion and a way to achieve success.

We continued training and learning from Evans for the next three months, in which time I got hooked. Shortly after, Evans was in a motorbike accident and passed away. God rest his soul in peace. Just like that, we lost our beloved teacher who inspired so many of us to become more than what we ever thought possible. He left a mark on my life, and I will be forever grateful for all he shared in the period of time that he was with us.

After a month of confusion and not knowing how or where to go from there, we got word about an upcoming yoga teacher training. We applied, and having come from Evan's outreach community, Job and I were given a straight pass in honor of our teacher.

Yoga was like a dream come true for me. It hit me and woke me up. It is through yoga that I became truly aware of what I could contribute to my life and the world around me. I began looking at things differently by asking what my contribution could be. I questioned my foundation and worked at making it better. I questioned some of my deep-seated beliefs about who I was and what I wanted in life. Through my physical practice, I experienced and witnessed my life outside the mat. The challenges in the pose were synonymous with the challenges in life. The sensations born of the physical exertion are the same as obstacles we come across off our mats. All these sensations have one characteristic—they keep rising and falling away as do life's challenges. I saw the lie in my life and the flaw in my story. I got in touch with the present through breathing, believing that nothing else mattered except this life force within me at that moment. I found that my position in life did not dictate who I am and who I wanted to be because the next moment would be different.

My advice now to you is to always be open and ready to see what is possible for you in every given moment. Embrace change in life and try not to be afraid of taking on new challenges and trying new things. Always search for the balance of both body and mind, equanimity.

You just might find your own "yoga."

The Impact of Yoga on My Life

When I first started practicing yoga, I was curious about why Swami insisted on yoga as a path to finding one's answers. I stayed alert during yoga class, mostly because I was a self-proclaimed fitness instructor who was looking at making a living out of the fitness industry. I immediately became captivated by the way the teacher taught the class. Being a self-taught acrobat turned "teacher," I was pretty good at poaching ideas from different sources, and quickly realized that I was going to take up yoga instruction. I listened carefully to the words of the teacher, it felt like he was talking to me.

One thing that stuck with me was the reference the teacher made about a physical pose mirroring our lives. He said, "consider that how you show up on your mat is exactly how you show up in your life." This statement was heavy, and I almost missed what the teacher meant, but I am glad that I got it. You see, your physical foundation equates to the foundation of anything you undertake in life, whether it is education, relationships, work, and career, or something else. I learned that the more grounded and connected I am to my "why," the more guarantee I will have of a good outcome. It took me a while to see its true application in life but when I did, it made a lot of sense.

This same principle applies to a building. The foundation of a building will determine how high it can be built and its durability. If you were to choose between sand and rock, you will with no doubt want to build your house on a rock and not on loose sand. These teachings have stayed with me for a long time and have guided me into significant teachings and milestones in my life ever since.

All these years as I worked as a professional acrobat in Kenya, I did not keep any records of my earnings or manage a budget. But how do you expect to make informed decisions without records and financial reports? You would think that this would be common sense, but not for me. Common sense is not very common after all. You see, subjects like Life Skills 101 are not taught in schools or in institutions often enough, my friends, at least not in the schools and institutions that I attended. And if they were, then they weren't drummed in well enough to have a lasting effect.

Without records, I was literally flying blind. My foundation was wobbly, it was like walking on water without a permit from Jesus. All I did was rely on a) luck, b) friends in high places, and c) managers and agents to find us work. I failed to see and understand the phrase "how you do anything is how you do everything." Even during rehearsals, where I thought I gave it my all, I came to realize I only did enough to secure a job and just enough to get paid. This is a sign of a not so strong a foundation, not connected to my "why!" Being blown around by the wind like a flag, I just swung to the tune. I got stuck in my comfort zone, dancing to the tunes of others and never taking charge and or accountability.

Never get too comfortable! Always seek to move out of your

comfort zone for that is where you will find growth.

This pattern continued for an entire twelve years. We did earn good money during some of the years. We'd end up spending most of it, if not all, by the time another job or gig came through. This happened to me again and again. A great proverb by Albert Einstein: "The definition of insanity is doing the same thing over and over again, but expecting different results." But we all get stuck at some point in life, I guess. We are all mad, only the degree differs!

What I discovered through yoga is how much of a visual learner I am. I learned to equate my physical yoga practice to my life outside the mat. Slowly and painstakingly I started to realize the practical steps that I needed to take to achieve the results I wanted. From this space, I created an inquiry around my life that then led to a new way of thinking. I minimized the "blame game" and realized that I had created and molded my life exactly the way it was. I had been playing the victim for a long time. Not just a victim of my circumstances, but a victim of my own making. I realized for the first time how I loved and bought into my own stories of why things did not happen for me the way that they happened for others.

This was my wakeup call, and I went from waiting for help from agents and friends and relying on luck, to taking action.

At the time, I had to find private classes that would help me make the transition from performing into teaching yoga. I worked hard as a teacher to gain experience and confidence. The most work had to be done on me. I didn't realize it's so much work, you know, working on me! I developed an understanding of how to be the best student that I could be, and how to show up fully in my own life. With this new revelation, somehow, I attracted people who were like-minded. I found a mentor through my affiliation with the Africa Yoga Project, the studio and organization that I give credit to for allowing me to become who I am today. My mentor's name is Suzie Newcome. Suzie took me through this very critical moment of self-realization and discovery. She helped me identify what would support and align with what I wanted in life. And how to drop everything else that did not serve me and my course or purpose. Yoga found me, I would say, at the right time in my life.

In Kenya, just like in many countries, I believe there are different classes or statuses. The rich, the middle class and the lower, poor class and slum dwellers, otherwise known in Kenya as ghetto peeps. In each category, there are things that are common and others that are regarded as strange, depending on where you fit in. A good example is the smoking of kaya, also called cannabis, weed or "the herb," as people from my locality would call it. To the high and upper-middle-class, kaya is a luxury. To the poor, it is a necessity. When life hits you so hard, you find a way to hide from it. It is a way of numbing out, as my teacher Baron Baptiste would say.

The rich and middle-class drink in bars and pubs, and the poor people's only options are local brew in a dingy bar or in homesteads. The preparation of local brew is not regulated, and the brew has been known to cause blindness and death. It comes from poor, "fake scientists" trying to make a quick buck without spending a lot of money. They experiment with chemicals, using poor human beings as guinea pigs.

Those of us who'd heard stories about this didn't take our chances with the local brew. As youths, we stuck with the herb that we believed to be pure and natural. We would smoke and listen to reggae music blasting through our ten-foot-by-ten-foot single rooms, and nobody would bother us. Depending on its quality and where it came from, we would choose the herb over food, even when it made us feel more hungry.

With the herb, we would drown our sorrows, numb ourselves, or simply knock ourselves out until we were hungry enough to go look for food. Baron understood that this is how lower-class people would roll. He also understood that this was the only way we knew how to handle life in these difficult conditions. It was Baron and Paige Elenson, the Director of the Africa Yoga Project, that understood the challenges of Kenya's youth and decided to provide free yoga to instill hope in those struggling with life's hardships. What we needed was somebody who would understand, and not condemn us; somebody who was willing to work with us and show us an alternative way as opposed to criticizing and labeling us as failures. Some say, "You look at someone the way he is, he becomes worse, and you look at him the way he should be, his potential is endless."

And so, together during our teacher training, we discussed the downside of the herb; the disadvantages of numbing out and how this stole from us instead of adding value to our lives. First, as an illegal drug in Kenya, it made us vulnerable and exposed to the wrath of the law. Second, when we smoked, hiding became our thing, and we would only associate with those whom we were comfortable with. This became a problem! We did not meet or want to meet people who had different opinions that would challenge our way of thinking. We did not challenge ourselves either. We became anti-social and very selective about whom we associated with. We became comfortable with our status. Tim Cork writes, "Comfort is our enemy. With comfort comes complacency." We got consolation by convincing ourselves that it was okay to be in this "class," negating our responsibilities and not being accountable for our actions and inactions.

Through our yoga teacher training, we learned about integrity, and how our words bind us. How nothing works without integrity. In simple terms, integrity is the power of a given situation, system or process. When lose integrity, there is a level of disfunction that costs us in terms of the results we hope for or expect. We spoke about how being true to others also means being true to ourselves. Staying away from that which does not serve us or conform to the laws of the land. In these discussions, we saw very quickly how the herb was working against us and not supporting our life goals. We saw how, for any advancement in life, there has to be some adjustment; learning, adapting, evolving and growing; this means change. Change is inevitable, negative or positive, it is bound to happen, but we can choose the direction. The choice is to either park on the roadside and watch others go by, or get on the highway of life and be the change that we want to see in our lives. I realized that we needed to choose between who we were and who we wanted to be for ourselves and for others.

This is how I started to peel away and eliminate the unhelpful layers in order to expose myself and see my situation for what it was. I was a fraud. I had lied to myself over and over and had gotten addicted to the lie. I said I wanted one thing but my actions said something else. Like wanting to be financially free and yet not keeping records, not budgeting, and completely losing stability in my foundation.

During the good times, I started keeping a consistent financial record and putting my goals down on paper. This was a good way to keep track of my progress and to develop a winning habit. I started making informed decisions, and the choices that followed came easy as information became available to me. This, as you can imagine, has brought my life to where it is today. I am headed far beyond where I was a few years back. I have made a great leap in a span of a few years; more than I had made in the many years since the beginning of my career. This is how beneficial yoga has been to me. It caused me to be open to learning, to be coached, and to teach. "When we teach, we learn twice." When we teach, we learn at a much deeper level. Be a teacher; it is a way of giving back and not holding back. Marianne Williamson wrote, "Your playing small does not serve the world. There is nothing enlightened about shrinking so that other people won't feel insecure around you."

Shine on my friend.

My Interpretation of Yoga

The word yoga in Sanskrit means to yoke, unite, or otherwise bring together the physical, mental, and spiritual or soul. When these three come together, we call it yoga. The above is the definition of yoga and this is my interpretation of it:

I have done yoga for the longest time, and maybe so have you. I didn't know it and might even have called it a different name. See, yoga is anything done physically with our whole being—our mind, body, and spirit. Most women do this when they cook family meals, wash dishes and perform other chores in the home. It is the same for men who perform activities that require the concentration of the mind and heart. Yoga is essentially cultivating this awareness so that it becomes second nature. It does not come overnight. It can, therefore, become a life goal and, with continued practice and persistence, a lifestyle.

Yoga is a journey of discovery through oneself to the self. You discover who you are and who you are becoming as you continue on this path as a student of life. In the Baptiste methodology of yoga, we study and practice yoga from three essential pillars.

Asana (physical practice), Inquiry, and Meditation. Through the physical practice, we build strength and stamina of the body and mind. This is the stamina and strength needed in your quest—a quest to liberate yourself from self-made shackles and limiting beliefs about who you are and what you can or cannot do.

It liberates you from the worldly attachments that cause you misery. It calls for awareness of our thoughts based on our sensations. It brings attention to how we act or react to these sensations that bring out our emotions. These emotions dictate the words, and the words inform our actions or non-actions. This integration of the whole is my understanding of yoga:

- Having a working knowledge of a concept or theory through experience.
- Being in touch with my physical self, through awareness of the sensations in the body, even the most subtle ones.
- Staying connected through breath and therefore the mind.

I believe that connecting these three aspects brings us closer to the highest self and purpose, the trinity of the mind, body, and spirit or soul.

An Inquiry, the second essential pillar, prods you to generate questions that inspire and challenge yourself. This helps bring alignment and attention to what you want to have happen and what is missing in your focus. It helps bring attention to your foundation and *your* "why"—why you do anything with the knowledge that your foundation is the key. The more rooted and grounded you are in your foundation, the more stable and profound the results. The Inquiry asks us how we show up in our lives, in the activities that we undertake with friends and or family, and whether we are contributing to or taking away from humanity.

The third pillar, Meditation, is a beautiful way of centering ourselves at any given time. We all know the benefits of concentrated effort and the theory of penetration. The smaller and sharper the tip, the easier it is to penetrate and vice versa. Meditation improves our concentration and slows our mind and our heart rate. With meditation, you can take away the mind's agitation and enter a calm state where you can focus on what is of the essence. With this, we can reduce stress-related issues in our lives. We can create more freedom in our way of being that is supportive of our chosen purpose and highest intentions. Meditation also can help bring intentionality in the things we do, so that we move away from acting by default into acting with purpose and intention. This is why yoga can only be a lifestyle and not something you simply engage in for short periods, because the results are lifelong.

Yoga has taught me a principle that has been mentioned by many writers and motivational speakers, including Mark Victor Hansen and Robert Allen in their book, *One Minute Millionaire*, and Earl Nightingale in his motivational talks. It is the principle of BE, DO, HAVE: that we attract that which we are and not necessarily what we want. I will give you a simple example using my next goal, a full side split, or Hanuman asana in Sanskrit. For me to achieve my goal, I will need to.

- **BE**:
  1. Someone who practices regularly.
  2. Someone who wants to know how muscles function.
  3. Someone who has a clear plan on how to work on the splits.
  4. Someone who has established metrics and habits that will keep him on track and focused.
  5. Someone who enrolls the help of a coach.

6. Someone who listens to instructions.
7. Someone who understands what needs to be done.

- **DO:**
1. Practice the splits.
2. Do the work or assignments I am given.
3. Do more than I am required to do.
4. Constantly thinks about my goal.
5. Do my part and do not meddle in other people's affairs.

If I BE and DO the above, I will HAVE what I want. I know it sounds simple, but it remains out of reach for many. That is why I say yoga is primarily a lifestyle: You are always learning and improving yourself day by day.

Yoga with African Traditions and Culture

The principle of yoga has been lost to a lot of people because they have not taken the time to investigate or understand it. There are a number of things that we might not agree with in yoga, and yet there are some that are totally acceptable and will conform to the natural laws of the universe. In fact, most do. Yoga is a way to approach human health in the most profound way—from the physical, mental and spiritual, although not necessarily religious. This approach has been studied by many teachers or sensei, gurus and yogis from all over the world, and they have come to the consensus that it is a beneficial practice for all to adopt.

When I look back at my own cultural traditions, some of the things I recall from the elders are similar to what yoga teaches us. I will use an example from the Luhya tradition that I come from. On the third day after circumcision, the circumciser comes back home to bless and offer guidance to the newly circumcised boy. The boy is covered in nothing but a blanket, sitting on a small stool by the door of his small hut facing outside. The boy sits tall and still, looking straight ahead, hands resting on his knees. Tapping the boy's shoulders with his special stick, the circumciser gives the boy a talk that guides him in his journey as a young adult. "Your heartbeat is strong; listen to it," he says. "It bears the strength of a man who stood the test of a knife. It will carry out the responsibilities of a man without blinking. The knife that you now hold, squeeze it tightly, it is a symbol of your transition from boyhood into adulthood. Feel the strength inside you as you squeeze on the handle of the blade. You are now a man old enough to plant a seed in a woman. Guard your ways, and do not find yourself in some other man's house or home. Stay firm in your feet and be grounded in the beliefs of our people and the traditions of our ancestors. Hold the respect of your home, your father and grandfather. Respect your elders and look to them for advice when unsure. Never deviate from the norms of our culture." We call this practice, "Khubita," and this, my friends, could be likened to guided meditation, and many other things that have been hailed by ancient yogis. Another example is the Maasai chanting, a practice that is common in many other tribes in Kenya as well. This custom is also similar to many different forms and styles of yoga.

Because of these strong similarities between our traditions and yoga, I think yoga as a physical practice should be encouraged in the institutional curriculum. Some people are more visual learners than others, including myself. Some vital life lessons could be delivered through a physical practice like yoga. Yoga brews consciousness in our daily thoughts, words, and deeds. It creates a space of inquiry around our thoughts and thought processes that are critical in forming the behaviors and habits that are forward-moving and supportive to all. James Allen in his book, *As a Man Thinketh*, says "People imagine that thought can be kept a secret, but it cannot; it rapidly crystallizes into habit, and habit solidifies into circumstance."

With this understanding we can listen for the thoughts and words that inform our actions, then we can get on the path of self-discovery in more profound ways. Yoga can help create this communal support and alliance that will make a difference in how we approach life. This, I believe, is the solution to uplifting many from the grassroots into a world of choice and personal power.

My Early Days in Yoga

Yoga is simple and reflects how the body is designed to move and operate. As a student, yoga gave me a new sense of awareness of my body. It brings breath and consciousness to major muscle tissues, and a chance to connect the mind and body. This is why yoga clicked for me. I was curious about the functions of a human body and the relationship between physical fitness and mindfulness. I remained open, emptied my plate, so to speak, and was ready for a fresh serving. I was willing to try a new approach to earning a living and to harnessing my true power, as I later came to realize. I understand that yoga might not be for everyone, and this is okay. We are all different and I respect the differences and uniqueness that we each represent. And yoga offers benefits far beyond the physical and spiritual, which can cause confusion. It is for this reason that I have chosen to stay out of any spiritual discussion in this book.

However, I will tell you more of what I have discovered along my path as a yogi looking for meaning and results in my life. I want to take you back to how yoga has improved my life. As a performing artist, my primary focus was to keep fit and be ready with my product, which was our performance. We did this with no trouble at all. Even when we had to work on empty stomachs, our focus on our goal kept us going. You see our goal, which remains the goal of many artists in Kenya, was to get a well-paying contract outside the country. Outside jobs paid more than local gigs for acrobats and dancers at the time. Performing arts in Kenya were seen as lowly ways of making money or making a living. Some people stereotypically believe that it is work only for the poor–"slum dwellers who have nothing else to do." The "nothing else to do" part is true to some extent, particularly when you look at the resources and options available to people from the lower class who have not had much of an education. Talent, except for sports, was looked down upon, and yet it is a trillion-dollar industry worldwide today.

Anyway, let me get back to my point. When we trained hard, our concentration was at the maximum, and after a few years of struggling, we made it. We took our shows everywhere, to whomever cared to see us, which included people on the streets. This earned us our very first gig outside the country as a group, and we were very happy. When I look back, I see that we succeeded in this aspect because we put in all the effort necessary, and it paid back.

As we moved into our next phase, having come from a background of scarcity and now suddenly into some cash, it threw us off guard for a while. Our expenses were all over the place. We purchased a lot of non-essential things. This dug into our pockets, leaving us dry and waiting for the next contract to come through. Clearly, we were not equipped to handle this new phase. It might be hard to imagine, but it took me close to eleven years in the industry to recognize this cycle and to start looking for a way out.

Some life lessons come to us in different ways; sometimes early, sometimes later, and at times after hitting rock bottom or after the near-death of a loved one or ourselves.

Mine happened when our firstborn daughter was two and our second baby was born. This is when I realized how helpless I could be as a father and as a husband. I slowly started looking for new ways to earn money and stop relying on acrobatic performing contracts, which had become few and far between. Maybe it was God's way, or the powers that be, deciding that it was time that I learned my lesson. As there were no more jobs coming in, it was around this time that I started getting into yoga. I spent a lot of my free time reflecting and asking what I was doing with my life. Incidentally, this was the one time that my wife expected results: food and money on the table, not thinking or reflecting. Her second pregnancy was the most difficult and nothing was working her way. She was stressed out. We quarreled almost every day, and even when we didn't, there was a "cold cloud–a cold war" in the air at all times.

"Your meditation sounds like a fantasy of dreamers, and we don't have that luxury," she said.

"Dreamers are the makers of this world, you know," I retorted with a growl too low to be heard. Rent was a problem and her wages were not enough. I could not afford to buy Pampers for my little girl; we had to use towels and second-hand napkins from Gikomba, the largest second-hand market in Nairobi. I sacrificed lunch and tried to eat very little at dinner to reduce my share and leave the rest for my wife and two babies. Sometimes, when I looked at them, I couldn't help but drop a tear. I kept thinking, why? Why me? I saw no way out and was growing more and more depressed.

This is the life I was living when I took on yoga, practicing, teaching and becoming a student of life. I was desperately searching for meaning in life and ways to become a good father and husband and an efficient provider for my family. I needed something, or someone to help ground me. I was flying high in my thoughts, in my head. But I had lost touch with the ground and the motivation to find my "why." Yoga revealed to me that there actually was something I could do, but first I needed to work on myself to be more accepting of where I was. I had to accept that it is painful and stressful, but I had to stay the path anyway. Acceptance is the very first step towards healing.

Before you set your GPS tracking device in your car, you have to key in your location. You need to know where you are coming from before you know where you are headed. Unfortunately in this phase of acceptance, nothing seems to be happening on the outside. There still is no money and no food on the table—in my case, only "air-burgers" and empty promises. And yet somehow that is when everything happens. Less is more; we say this all the time in yoga and in many other platforms. See, it is at this point of acceptance that we start the forces of change within us. We free ourselves from our shackles and brace ourselves for a flight of self-discovery. With self-acceptance, we acknowledge our past and agree to put it behind us. Now, the slate is clean, we have erased our blame game, excuses, and the concerns that hold us back. Now we are free to act and to be who we want to be.

The art world in Kenya did not pay well, but there were still a few places that wanted entertainment. These gigs provided a small income, which allowed me to support my family and push forward through the days. I had hopes that December, high season for artists in Kenya, would bring in more contracts, but for some reason that year it wasn't the case. Things were terrible and I felt the world was collapsing around me. I once read somewhere that misfortunes don't come in a single dose. Once they start, they come in a series. It was never more true for me than in this period.

By December tenth we had only managed a handful of gigs landing us each with 5,000 shillings, or fifty dollars, in our group of six people. So, you can imagine my excitement when on December 11th, I received a call that landed us a gig outside of town towards the central part of Kenya on the 25th of December 2012. This was supposed to be our season finale, and we had high hopes that we would end the year in good spirits, and with a generous amount of cash in our pockets.

Mukutano Junction

The much anticipated day had come: We, the Zamasimba Acrobats, arrived from the city. We were on time for the opening show scheduled for 1:00 pm at Elegance Gardens in Sagana, on the way to Nyeri.

"Zamasimba is an acrobatic group all the way from Nairobi. They have trained and worked together since 2001. For eleven years they have traveled the world with their mesmerizing show and today we are happy to have them grace us with their awesome acrobatic shooow!!" announced the emcee of the day, Mr. Mwano. "Zamasimba is much bigger than the five represented in this book, we have silent members just so you know!"

The audience was filled with churchgoers and people celebrating Christmas, looking for a place to hang out with their families on this memorable day. Despite the audience being a bit reserved at first, the show was a success and the crowd quickly warmed up. It all went well, and we had so much fun, especially with the young members of the audience.

Eventually, it was time for us to wind up and leave; we had

a long journey back home. We said our quick goodbyes to the host DJ, emcee, and the management crew. We promised to come back again on the 31st of December for another performance, as if it were up to us.

Out on the road our group, Mathu, Obach, Karanja, Job and I, waited for a matatu, that was heading back to the city. Matatu, as they are known in Kenya, are a common public means of transport, usually via a small fourteen-seat van or a minibus.

Mathu was one of the new members of Zamasimba. A strong character, tough, and quick to anger. Obach was the youngest of the group. A good boy, he was very loyal with sharp reflexes, and a good team player. Karanja was an age-mate of Mathu, quiet and reserved, though he spoke his mind. He would shy away from any confrontation. Job was a close friend and pioneer member of Zamasimba. One of the old lions in the den, he is sober, rational and can keep his head even under pressure. Then there was me: The oldest lion in the park! Just kidding, no was not.

We eventually flagged one of the Nissan matatus and asked a very specific question to the driver: "*Unafika Nairobi tao, ama wewe ni wa kukwama njiani?*" ("Is this an express service to the city or not?")

The conductor responded nicely, "*Aah mimi ni wa Nai direct hii ni nganya mpaka kati kati ya jiji.*" ("I am going directly to the city; this is a new van, it goes to the city center.") All five of us boarded the matatu to Nairobi in good spirits, chit-chatting away as we got in.

Makutano is a market center at a junction on the road to Embu/Meru and the route to Karatina/Nyeri. We arrived at this point and both driver and conductor decided it wasn't worthwhile for them to continue on to Nairobi. They instead decided, against their word, to make a U-turn and head back. Obviously, we were a little upset by this change of plans, although it was expected. Somewhere along the way the conductor had hinted that it did not matter if they continued, as long as we got to the city–that it made no difference to him or us whether he drove us there or found us another matatu to do the same. This, of course, made a lot of sense from a business perspective, but it was an inconvenience to us and broke his promise.

The public transport industry in Kenya is unregulated, especially the matatus. The sheer lack of courtesy and customer satisfaction can be worrying. Their focus is to maximize the present with no concern for tomorrow.

At the junction, where we had alighted for the changeover. Mathu, Obach and the conductor argued as to whether to let him go or to hold him until he paid the next vehicle to take us to the city. You see, it was Christmas day, and there are fewer vehicles plowing the route to Nairobi on a big holiday. Further, makangas have a habit of giving you change that will not be accepted by other matatus, and guess who pays the difference? You.

While still arguing, one of the resident makangas joined in the discussion, but he did not wait to understand what the argument was all about. Instead, the newcomer stretched his hand and took the five-hundred-shilling note held by our makanga. This made Mathu very angry, and you didn't want Mathu to get angry! He thought it was bad enough for this rude, new entrant to budge into the conversation, but to take the money—it was too much!

Mathu shoved him a little and this guy pushed him back. Opportunity finds a window. Before he knew it, *phaaat*, a straight punch landed squarely on his cheek. "Ooh oh, what the hell," was all I could manage to say. I had not been expecting a fight. So, in my humblest character, I moved fast to try and defuse the situation before it got out of hand. Job and Karanja joined as we tried to block Mathu and Obach from the confrontation, but we were gradually attracting a crowd of men from around the terminus.

It quickly became apparent that we had no control over the growing crowd. Most of the men were drunk, hungry for blood, and did not listen to anything we said. We tried to avoid more physical confrontations, but it was too late. In the span of about three minutes, the crowd had grown to almost fifteen people. One of the local guys told me to get my guys out before it became worse.

"*Wanakuja wengi na miti, endeni sahii*," he said. ("More are coming with huge sticks; you should leave now while you can.") He was begging us to leave.

I tell you, everything was happening so fast it was crazy.

Just as I got my guys to start leaving, a man pulled hard on my bag. He was visibly drunk and threw a punch at me. Instinctively, I ducked and reacted with one of my own. This sent him down, still clutching onto my bag, dragging me down with him. He was as heavy as a full bag of potatoes. Within a few seconds, there were three more descending on me, kicking. When Mathu saw this, he came back with an iron rod and hit one of them across the back. The man fell flat on the ground with a thud. I quickly fought my way out of the small group before the rest of the crowd caught up.

It was then that we realized we had to run for our lives. All I could think of was a saying in Swahili, "*miguu niponye*." ("Save me, my legs.") We ran like hell, covering a distance of no less than two hundred meters Olympic style, except that we had significantly sized bags with our performance gear on our backs. These guys were persistent and followed us into a bar compound where we thought we'd be safe for a while as we strategize our next step. Wrong move!

It was here that we made the big mistake which I will never

forget. I cautioned my boys not to be so fast in running away since we were dealing with locals, and they would surely know where we might surface if we took a matatu to Nairobi. They could waylay us. I have never been so wrong in my life. I should have followed the other guys' advice. One wanted us to run to the back and climb over the back wall. While we took that little time contemplating our next move, the goons had gathered and came at us with the renewed force of the mob. We made a run for it out through the back entrance and over the wall. Halfway up the wall, I noticed Job was not with me.

Soldiers don't leave their fellow men behind.

Little did I know, the paramilitary training still had a grip on me. It was the wrong application of that principle if you ask me. The best solution would have been to run away with the boys and go to the police. I wasn't in my best mental state, then, was I? There is a comedian who once highlighted the difference between a John White and Wambilianga from Africa.

"On seeing a leopard, Wambilianga screams out loud, Leopard! and runs for his dear life. John White, always the adventurer, goes, hey kitty kitty….hrrrrrrrr, and John gets torn to pieces by the leopard."

Here, I was being John White. I knew what the mob is capable of but some stupid voice in my head told me they would listen to reason. I have never been so wrong! I couldn't leave Job behind, so I climbed back down still holding, unconsciously, one of the one meter long, limbo metal rods that we use in our show. Talk of coming to a peace treaty with a cocked gun in hand! I should have set it aside. This little miscalculation, plus hesitating going over the wall almost cost us our lives. The mob had caught up with us and demanded that we follow them out, threatening the management not to get involved or they would burn down the premises.

The management chose to comply.

Well, this was the end of sanity, my friends. Everything that I had ever learned about diplomacy and how to apply it did not work. Job tried desperately to drum sense into the local guys' heads because they spoke the same language, but nothing worked. They kicked, punched and hit us with sticks. They kept asking where the other three were, and we kept repeating the same answer over and over: "They are back there and should be coming soon." It was a white stupid lie that we told so we didn't seem rude by keeping quiet. When you are scared you say all sorts of things, I tell you. I don't know why we said it. We should have said something clever like, "They've gone to the police." That should have scared them a little. But no.

They led us back in the direction we had run from. Along the way, the number of men kept increasing. Now we were surrounded by a crowd of about thirty to forty people. The problem with such a crowd is that you cannot communicate effectively with anyone. Believe me, every fifth, sixth and seventh guy will not hear you, and nothing will stop him from exercising his manliness and unleashing the beast inside him.

Some would launch flying kicks that would either miss us so terribly that you'd want to laugh, especially when they get one of their own. Then you would remember, "Ooh that kick was aimed at me." Before the thought was finished, he came back at you with a devil blow right to your nose. Then stars were all you'd see. "I must be on my way to the moon, or is it my imagination playing tricks on me?" The 21st-century astronaut with no gear? Hmm for a moment there, I was dazed. Lucky for them I didn't faint; they could have had some weight to bear! As if that would matter.

As they continued to march us on, they kept discussing amongst themselves the best place to finish us off. They came to a halt right outside a shop where there was another small crowd. These people couldn't say or do anything to save us. This was when I decided to make peace with God and to say my last prayers. So many thoughts went through my head: thoughts of what an awful way to die, thoughts of this fateful day, and the events in this whole season. I thought it was my time and that God had decided to punish me for all my wrongdoing on earth. My children's lives flashed before me, and the thought of not having a chance to redeem myself as a father broke me. My two-year-old had accidentally burnt herself with hot tea in the kitchen just the day before, and my youngest did not even know me yet. She was only nineteen days old and had just come home from the hospital that very day, the 25th of December, 2012. After being in an incubator for a week due to premature birth, finally, she could come home. She couldn't make out faces yet. What if she saw my face, then? Can you imagine? A one-eyed face with a deep cut on the nose, swollen cheeks? She would be haunted for life. Imagine when your kid sees you for the first time and her first impression of you is of a vampire? Horror? You are a horror to your own child. So much for fatherhood, huh! Good thing she was only nineteen days old—she wouldn't know better.

By then we were bleeding profusely. My t-shirt was drenched in blood and more was dripping from my nose and a cut just under my right eye. My friend Job was not doing any better. He had a deep cut into his left elbow, oozing blood like a punctured packet of milk, and another cut on his forehead. He had persisted, talking. But he was giving up. I urged him on and told him not to give up and to keep talking even when they seemed not to listen. The relentless talk did help to an extent.

At this point, you might be wondering why I was not contributing to the discussion. You see, this was a time in Kenya when a sect called the Mungiki were on the rise. They belonged to the Kikuyu tribe, which is Job's tribe. These guys were like a rebel army and they were wreaking havoc, mostly in the central province where we were. They discriminated against any tribe that did not speak their language. They were known to maim, and even kill people, who did not belong to their tribe or did not conform to their beliefs and principles. I happened to come from a different tribe, and that alone would have been reason enough to kill me and Job for his association with me.

Eventually, they sat us down on the unpaved road. This is how thieves, robbers, and rapists in central Kenya and other places are treated. Whenever a crowd makes its victims sit down, it marks their last moments alive. Lynching follows, and rubber tires are put around them, petrol poured and a match dropped.

I believe this was our mob's plan, but they did not find tires fast enough. They had decided to kill us right there, if they had the tires. Instead, they continued clobbering us from all directions and with everything you can think of. Some broke the nearby fence posts to use as weapons. Luckily for us, one of the posts was too heavy to wield easily, so one guy struggled with it. And that was when an involuntary scream escaped Job, "*Wooi*, don't kill us!" The guy dropped the post and it bounced towards me. I raised my hands over my head, and luckily, held the weight with my hands. Somebody stepped forward with one of the metal bars we used in our show for limbo. He lifted it over his head, aiming for my mine. I blocked it again with my hands. The man raised the bar again, but thank God, it was hollow, so it warped into a V-shape upon impact. He stopped, feeling good about his work.

The beating went on until a God-sent rumor rippled through the crowd: that the police were close by and heading in our direction. This scared our assaulters enough to release us, but carefully enough so that we couldn't see where they ran. Two of our attackers led us towards the main road and waved down a matatu coming from Embu. They gave the driver instructions to take us away from the spot immediately. The matatu driver sped off with us in a panic.

After we had driven a safe distance, we told the matatu driver to hang on for a minute as we had three friends still in hiding. As we waited, the driver gave us an account of his own experience. He had been through the same situation with people in the same town. He offered to hold on as we tried to reach our three missing comrades on the phone. It turned out that Obach, the youngest of us, had made it back to the main road at the Makutano junction. He'd changed his shirt and lowered his cap to conceal his identity. He made it home safely in two hours.

We eventually located Mathu and Karanja and headed to Thika, from where we took another matatu to Nairobi looking like a bunch of guys from a scene in the post-election violence that took place in 2007-08, in which hundreds of innocent Kenyans lost their lives.

This is a story that the pioneer members of the Zamasimba Acrobats will never forget, and for Job and me, a close shave.

The Shepherds

Three shepherds are looking after their sheep around Mai Mahiu, a market center along Nakuru-Nairobi highway. The shepherds and the sheep cross the road as a big trailer truck approaches from the slopes. Roughly one hundred head of sheep are spread over a distance of about twenty yards. Unfortunately, the shepherds leave it to the truck driver to decide the fate of their sheep, and the truck smashes right into the herd just as they are crossing. The sheep became confused, and the shepherds run around, picking up the dead and half-dead sheep, forgetting all about guiding the living sheep out of the road. The driver, having made the decision to keep driving, bumps and shoves more sheep off the road. In their pain and grief, the shepherds get trapped in the moment and forget to help the alive sheep to safety. Silly herdsmen? Hmm, maybe not.

What is your trap? What is the one thing that is making you so panicked that you don't see anything beyond it? What is this one thing that is holding you back from assessing the big picture, from doing the things that will lead you or others to safety? It could be your anger, like it was for Zamasimba Acrobats when we got trapped in Makutano junction on that fateful day in December. "It could be money, it could be your ideas about happiness and if you could just let go, then you could experience real happiness. It could be your ideas about how your partner looks, acts and smells like that is trapping you," writes Prince E.A.

We all get trapped by one thing or another. The first thing to do is to accept what has happened and take the next step forward. Let experience teach you. Use your experiences to learn from the mistakes that you've made, and share widely so that we can all continue to grow. Learn to let go of all the pain, hatred, and the anger that is trapping you.

This incidentally happens through self-awareness and identifying the sensations in your body. They inform your moods and spirit or attitude. Make a point to move away from the state that is trapping you; trapping more sheep, like in the shepherds' story, and forgoing safety for all of us in danger in the Zamasimbas' case. The more you hold onto your anger, the more hurt you bring to yourself and others. Notice your traps and let go of them all. This way you can create more space for peace, love, and community.

Yoga changed my way of living and interacting with people. I was stuck for years in my career as an acrobat and never took steps forward. I lacked what you might call "make-it-happen" power. I needed to get off my seat, market and showcase our product more effectively, and get out of my comfort zone. I managed to start this process after opening my mind to yoga. The yoga approach and philosophies made all this doable, but not obvious. My journey had only just begun.

On so many occasions I had hundreds of excuses for why something was not happening for me. I never stopped to ask myself what my contribution to the situation was. Contribution towards a certain goal is what counts as effort. What was I doing to move the log or obstacle out of the way, or better yet, to move around it?

In yoga, we learn to flow like water. Water does not struggle to make its way. It simply flows downwards, never up. When it comes across an obstacle, it moves around it. It may need to change course, but it doesn't matter, it will always stay the course.

Be soft to life and life will be soft to you. Keep contributing through your full participation and resourcefulness. Keep moving forward and let all the traps and distractions fall on the wayside. Draw your mat and keep your focus within the bubble of your mat and on your breath.

My Lie

I call it my lie because I have chosen to take ownership of it. I had been holding it close to my heart and living this lie for the longest time. I said and thought about this lie so many times that it became true.

My lie was that I was born in an underprivileged home. I always compared myself with those around me and saw myself as one of the unlucky ones, and one of the unloved. This lie had a big impact on my life, mostly negative—from my education, where I changed schools seven times in my nine-year period of primary education and in my childhood where I was raised by my grandma. None of that is bad; the bad part was just what I made it mean.

My mother was a primary school teacher and requested to be relocated from one school to the other several times. As I grew up, my grandma needed someone to live with and help with the farm work. As a young relative and one of the oldest grandsons, I was the perfect candidate. My grandma was a caring, loving, tough lady, and I received tough love. I can tell you now that I am who I am because of the good values she instilled in me.

I was managing my grandma's small farm of six acres by the age of eleven. I milked three to five cows every morning at 5:00 before heading to school at 7:00. I would do the same in the evening after making my forty-five-minute journey home on foot without shoes. Over the weekends I would take the animals to a nearby forest to graze and be gone for the whole day, just like somebody working a nine to five office job. The cycle continued day in and day out. In eighth grade, I took my encyclopedia, (a collection of books in all subjects in the Kenyan primary education curriculum) with me to the forest, as that was the only time I had to study. I scored average in my finals and went to an average high school that was about a two-and-a-half to three-hour-walk from home. It was this childhood, and a few other events in my life, that solidified my lie and cemented my belief that I was not lucky or loved.

Children can grow up with a certain perspective on life. A lot of things that I did back then were informed by my experience. I survived and had to work hard because I believed that is how life is meant to be. When I missed an opportunity to do something I wanted, I told myself I wasn't meant for it in the first place. I did not see myself as deserving of anything. Occasionally, I proved myself wrong by achieving good grades in college, scoring best in drills, or having the guts to choose a paramilitary college where I didn't have to bother anyone with fees. I entered a college meant for underprivileged youths who could not afford college fees. The college is sponsored by the government and in return, students pay the government through service to the nation. The service runs between eighteen months to two and a half years, after which students undertake their course of choice within the provision and are discharged from the service on completion. I wanted to protect myself from other people; I wanted to reduce my dependency on others. I wanted to prove that I could do it, that I was not so broken. My elder brother and sister were struggling through college, and I did not wish the same for me. So, I made decisions that avoided my getting hurt or being in other people's debt. This lie held me back, and it wasn't until I confronted this ghost from my past, understanding what my lie was, that I was able to unchain myself.

This is a foundational principle in yoga. Understanding that my lie is the story I tell myself about what happened in my life—what I made it mean and my interpretation of what happened. I had a very good story. In fact, I came to realize that we all have good stories about what happened to us in our pasts. However, the past is gone, and the future is created effectively by being present and understanding that each moment allows us to build our future. It is thus important to identify, revise and evaluate our stories again and again: to point out the facts, drop off any emotional attachments, and see what remains.

Allow me to share one other anecdote that was the root of my lie about not being loved. Back in 1987, my grandma was moving from where we were staying in a marketplace to a farm. We had managed to shift most of the belongings, but not all. Some six of twenty-four heads of cattle were still up in the mountains. Everybody in the extended family had been invited to the new house. All my uncles, aunts, and cousins came, but someone had to stay up in the mountains to look after the remaining cows and property. We had a worker, but granny would not leave the worker alone. Somebody from the family had to be there, and guess who that was? Me! I was eleven years old and was told to stay behind to look after the home and cattle while my siblings and cousins had all the fun. This was a blow that I never reconciled with. It was around Christmas time, and on the 24th of December I came down from the mountains to bring a few other things that were needed in the new home. I saw all my cousins playing, and I desperately wished that I could stay. But I couldn't. My grandma was quick to point out that since I was walking, I needed to get going before it got too late. I left with tears in my eyes, thinking she must really hate me to send me away from all this. I thought I was an outcast. No one liked me. My lie was planted, and from then on circumstances just made my lie more evident and worse.

Years later, through yoga, I was able to separate the story from the facts. I realized how much trust my grandma had in me. She entrusted her property and wealth in my hands, as young as I was because I was the best suited. She loved me a lot to do this. She also loved her animals, and I now see how you can't entrust something so precious to someone you don't like or trust.

This newfound clarity gave me so much room and space to appreciate all the things that she has done for me and how she loved me. I was so blinded by my lie that I had missed seeing how much she adored and loved me for who I was. But to realize this I had to accept that I was living a lie. I had to accept that I was looking at life from a different angle and that is all there is.

Acceptance is a gift we need to give to ourselves often. I needed to close this cabinet of files from my past so that they would stop spilling into my future; to give me space for a new and powerful future for myself and for all those that I care about.

It has been proven that 86 percent of self-talk is negative. This was exactly the case for me. This self-talk or internal conversation, when undistinguished, is taken as "me" talking, and as "me" saying what is true, what is possible and what isn't. Distinguished, it is simply a voice—a voice I must learn to live with, but ignore when I can, because it is not going anywhere soon. Discovering for myself the impact of my internal dialogue allowed me to be fully present and to listen. Creating this distinction was imperative for my forward movement. It gave me so much peace.

What is your lie?

Going beyond this called for more than listening to myself. By practicing yoga, being around others and sharing stories, I acquired insight into other people's lives and discovered how so many of us have the same ghosts holding us back from accessing who we truly are and reaching our potential. By listening, reading yoga journals and other inspirational books, and attending forums, the curtains started lifting. Little by little the light shone into my space and the shade receded. The shade in this context was my comfort zone. I realized that I had been very comfortable thinking that life would just keep happening, that I just needed to take it as it comes, blow after blow. But suddenly, I had the profound realization that I was in command; that the power rested in my hands to mold myself into who I wanted to be, both for me and for others. I began to understand what my contribution to the world had been, and what I wanted it to be. It is a full-time job changing oneself, and I learned that I had to work systematically and patiently to get the results that I wanted in life.

I have had so many excuses. I was born poor. I was unlucky. I was not well equipped to handle the test of life. But in the end, who really is? This voice in my head with all these excuses was disempowering, to say the least. This conversation has an impact on my life, and recognizing that this internal dialogue shapes all that I consider being true, which is based on the past, is key. The lie that I tell myself informs my interpretation of what happens to me in the real world. I experience it, I hear it, and I see evidence that cements and justifies my lie. My lie is based on history. Knowing that, I now hold the reins and can remold myself into the person I want to be. Confronting my past, closing it down, and making a choice to move on has been my biggest lesson.

The System Doesn't Define You

I believe that over history, two systems. The education system and the post-education system have been misunderstood or misused to define people. I also believe that in order to work within any system, we must understand why it was put in place, and how to use it as it was designed.

The Education System:

The education system in Kenya is mandated by the Kenyan Institute of Curriculum Development. It is centered on providing high-quality education, because education provides the highest return of any social investment and is key to breaking the cycle of poverty. It is known that empowering young people with knowledge and applicable skills fosters informed thinkers who understand their basic human rights and are capable of shaping the success of their family's health and wellbeing.

The objective of the education system is to 1) equip students so that they are strong, competent people who maximize their household resources in the informal economy (e.g. agriculture, small business development, and animal husbandry activities), 2) equip learners with employable skills to enter the workforce, and 3) academically prepare students for acceptance into post-secondary programs.

My story:

Back in school, I wanted to become an engineer of some sort. Teachers assured us that if we did not put the required amount of time and energy into our studies, that it would affect us for years to come. Most of us listened but didn't quite connect with that on a practical level. Teachers said education will inform the path we take, which I believe is very true.

In school, we all did our best, but I missed the mark by a few points and labeled myself a failure. Jim Rohn, is his book, *Leading an Inspired Life*, asks, "Is the best you can do, all you can do?" He thinks not, and I would totally agree with him. Rohn says if "you took a rest and came back to it, you could do some more." I wish I had had a second chance at my exams. I am sure I would have done better. It was only later that I came to learn that if I had connected my goals with an action plan early enough I would have had good results.

Back at home, it was worse for me. I had been raised by my grandma, partly because my mum, as a single parent, had struggled a lot and needed help raising six kids, and because my grandma needed someone to help on the farm and stay with her. This posed a lot of challenges in my study life. I tell you one thing, though, adversity is a great teacher. I learned very quickly that when you are raised in such an environment you don't have the luxury of failing. I remember a conversation with one of my uncles so vividly: He emphatically told me I had let them down as a family. Having been born from a female in their home (his sister), I was practically an outsider.

"All you have brought us is a shame," he said. "No single boy in this family has missed entry to university. How could you not recognize your status and worked hard enough to earn a scholarship? A scholarship would have been your only chance as your mother could not afford it even if you had good grades. Now, it is even worse because you did not even make the cut for any campus."

I was devastated and broken. I felt the blood drain from my face, my facial skin felt heavy and saggy. Tears ran down my cheeks, and I let my eyes close for a moment in the hopes of closing out the blurry vision of my own life. In my mind, I had lost it all, and that left me not valuable anymore, not ever. It was like something precious being pulled away from you, but you are so powerless, lacking the strength to reach out and make a scratch on its surface before it is completely taken away. I felt cheated, robbed of my life and dumped. With my eyes on the ground, feeling beaten, I walked away, coiled and shrunk like a bird that had been rained on. If I was a dog, I would have had my tail between my legs. Life was over for me, or at least it felt that way. That night, I contemplated taking my own life. That rope that I had used to tie up the new goat sounded like a good idea and a perfect way to go!

No, I did not take it that far, even though I stayed in the dark barn for the longest time with my dog, Simba. I didn't leave until my grandma sent for me, and even then, I did not want to go into the house. But it was getting so cold that I had no choice. I slept on an empty stomach that night. The following morning, I decided to go visit my mum. I felt unwanted, not loved and completely rejected. This all fed right in with my lie. I needed someone to reassure me of why I had to live on, and my mother did. We all need support, and sometimes it is just another shoulder to lean on, to listen to our anguish.

Be there for others and they will be there for you.

The system, by now, had made me into who I was. I saw myself as worthless in the eyes of the system. In front of my uncle and my teachers in the school, I felt like a complete failure because of the meaning I gave to my uncles' and my teachers' approach. Looking back now, I see that they wanted nothing but the best for me. Sometimes, when we listen to people, our interpretation is flawed, totally different from what they actually mean. It is therefore important to ask them to clarify what they've said or mean, and to take time to separate our story from the facts; to separate our story from the ego. The ego wants us to create a good story that makes us look good. The fact is, failure does not happen in one swoop, but rather in a series of small failures over time. If I had been willing and present enough to recognize my small failures along the way and found a way to learn from them, there is a chance that I could have done well and avoided failing my final exam.

You own your successes and failures. Learn from them and create a better chance and a better life for yourself.

Small gains and small failures:
Thought = feeling = action = results
Thought + Action = Results
Example goal: Pass my final exams
Feeling: Pride, sense of belonging, confidence
Action: Study (plan/schedule), strategy
Results: Success

Small gains: "*Kidogo kidogo hujaza kibaba*" is an African proverb that means "Bit by bit, the basket fills up."

Compound interest: Every time I follow my program as I have designed it, I become more knowledgeable in the subjects, producing great results, establishing a routine and learning all that I need to scale and sustain it.

As I grow and continue repeating this process, I have built my "principal" and "accrued interest." Now, I can generate more interest. Once I have established myself and demonstrated consistency, more opportunities come my way: new study content, exposure opportunities, people willing to partner with me and help. I make a small gain towards my goal. It's called compound interest and it works in life as well as for saving money.

Small failures: Anytime I miss studying as planned, I make a small hole out of my container of success; in other words, I step away from my goal. I have deducted from my account of success. This will accumulate to become my setback, and my eventual failure to reach my goal.

Without connecting these two principles of thought and action, success will remain elusive.

Take the example of a container that needs filling water as the goal. Success is measured by filling the container with water. It is designed to have an inflow and an outflow. The inflow could be equated to the number of small wins in your quest for success in your education life or whatever your goal is. The outflow indicates the number of small failures.

In this context, success becomes a simple mathematical equation. Inflow should always be greater than outflow. If X is inflow—the input of energy, effort, dedication, devotion, sacrifice, etc.—and Y is outflow—drainage, energy spent, minimal effort, less of anything and everything—then S is the achievement of the goal.

The formula of success:
$$X > Y = S$$

If the inflow of small gains remains relatively high in comparison to the outflow, we will be safe and successful.

The system is not meant to put boundaries as to who we can

or cannot be. The truth is, it doesn't do this, even if we think it does. Our perception is faulty. It is not meant to define us as people who pass exams, but rather people who are knowledgeable about certain life principles. When we study in schools, most of us study to pass exams. However, we should instead study to gain skills and knowledge to further our interests. And how do we do that? By seeking to understand the concepts as opposed to cramming and reciting for the final exam. If and when we understand the concepts, or the "why," we will be set on a different plane.

The objective of the system is to teach somebody to work their way out of their negative thoughts and suggest the right action for achieving the results they want. The underlying word is discipline; to maintain a chosen routine to create great habits that will help bring your dreams closer. Like Tim Cork says in his book *G3*, "Great habits create great success. These habits must become a daily ritual."

Training as acrobats was an uphill task and required a lot of patience and dedication. The results appeared much later, just like study and exam preparations during school. Our training program was tedious, and we had to keep at it for six months and more. We had to learn how to use preparation, good planning, and repetition to create habits that would help us become successful. John Dryden says, "First we make our habits and then our habits make us."

If students understood that the system does not define who they are as a person—that instead it is a strategic process of repetition to create habits that will enable them to access their true power—then they would receive more intentional and focused results.

Trevor Noah writes in his book, *Born A Crime,* about how many black people in South Africa internalized the logic of apartheid and made it their own. That is, they remained self-oppressed way after the oppression period. Let's look at another example of how Indians tamed their elephants. A young elephant is tethered with a chain to a tree. They are restrained until they become used to their new home. After this process, the elephant does not move far from the tree even after it is released, because it thinks it is still tethered and on chains.

Do not agree to be tamed or restrained by the system, as it is meant to give you freedom. What you know liberates you, and what you don't know holds you back. Try something new every day, especially something that scares you, and watch yourself grow.

As a society, we are so much more than the system. We make the system as opposed to the system making us. "What else is possible for me?" should be our focus, with the idea that what is possible is sometimes far beyond what we can see. We must harness the power of believing in the unseen before it manifests itself.

Academic achievements are very important as they define our path as a scholar, and everybody should strive to make it to the highest level of education possible for them. And, what we learn in the process accounts for so much more. We are continually practicing habits that will sustain us on the outside. If by bad luck, you take a wrong turn and fall into a ditch, you are the only one who can initiate the rescue process. If you don't call out for help when you need it, you will stay trapped.

After my uncle berated me, for example, I spoke to my mum. "All will be well my son," she said. It was all that I needed to hear. It was like magic. I felt so much better.

The curriculum provides you with the necessary tools to understand, accept and create solutions to mitigate what we call bad situations in life. Practical application of thought and action equals good results. True intelligence is understanding how to use the knowledge to help yourself and others.

You have got to be hungry, perhaps, before you take action and apply relevant knowledge. "Intelligent people are action-driven," says Tim Cork. Nothing happens until you take action. Be persistent in following your study timetable and action plan, and be good to others so that you do not waste time on trivialities. Great results are eminent when you follow your action plan. This is what you learn from the system.

Essentially, the system is meant to prepare us for life after school and what to expect outside the walls of schools and institutions. The system is only relevant to the point where it addresses what is real on the outside and directly impact who we are willing to become to achieve our goals. It instills the discipline and habits that we are willing to learn to become the person that wins. The system demands that we be successful.

After school or post-education system:

The system outside school is a continuation of what is started in class. In this digital era, if you did not go through campus or college, things tend to become tricky for you. Employers are looking for the most academically qualified candidates they can find. The less academic qualifications you have, the less you are paid. It does not matter how experienced you are; the first question is what degree or diploma do you hold? If you have none, you are paid peanuts in comparison with your counterpart who has no experience but who has the papers. These people end up becoming your superiors and oversee you on a job, even when you can teach them how to do it. Before you realize how futile it is to fight the system you will have wasted a lot of time, as I did. You end up struggling and living an unsatisfied and unfulfilled life of a low achiever. You become a complainer, living a victim's way of life. When complaining is the order of the day you don't realize that the more you do it, the more you attract the situations that will make you complain. This creates a never-ending cycle of events that are energy-draining and take you many steps away from your goals.

This realization came alive to me in yoga. My yoga teacher, Paige Elenson, and Baron Baptiste have drummed into me the essence of being in the present. They made me aware of how I must show up in anything I do and how important it is to capture the essence of what is happening right now in life, and not just letting it flow by. This, they said, will lay the foundation for knowing what actions to take and what stories to drop. These are universal principles that work, whether you know them or you don't. Your attitude will make you see it or not see it. Earl Nightingale in one of his audio talks says, "The word 'attitude' has been called the most important word in the world, and I believe that."

Something that people forget when they talk about working hard is the input. They think the input is only digging more into the material they learn; the sciences and art subjects or the different courses in their careers. What they forget is the addition of the most important word; attitude. Your attitude is your greatest asset. Attitude towards your plan of action will determine the kind of results you get. This is true whether you are in America, Europe, Asia or Africa. Ten percent is what happens to you, 90 percent is your attitude. You are the reason for your success and your failure.

"The most successful people in life are usually the biggest failures. They make lots of mistakes. They learn what works and what doesn't work and get better through that experience." says Tim Cork. The moment you realize this very important lesson in life—not just in school or an institution—you become a winner headed towards creating the kind of life you envisioned for yourself.

This is the starting point, as everything else tends to fall into place as you continue with a positive attitude in pursuing your goals and dreams. The right attitude and discipline in creating great habits is the one thing the system is meant to create in you. What you get out of the system equals your input in terms of effort and time. To provide a system that works for many, unfortunately, it also means the system will not spoon-feed you. It is not tailor-made to individuals. It is generalized, and that is where "you do you."

You create your own way of studying or your own contributions, however that might look. The system as it is created does not give. What we give to the system is what comes back twofold. Good teachers and facilitators will not give us this. What they do is create an enabling environment for you to get the concept and understand the implications. Good employers and organizations are the same. It's about the choices that you make as a person. Life is about choices. Your attitude is a choice. Choose wisely. Choose an attitude that serves you and your direction in life. And remember, if you choose to be cynical and negative, life will be cynical and negative towards you.

The system is a starter program for you to see and recognize what you want in life and how to go for it. You are an informed individual and you need to identify yourself as such. An informed person makes informed decisions and choices about their lives. They try not to get stuck in their stories, seek to understand the cause and effect, and make choices to move on. Self-victimization is a trait of low achievers and the poor. In this context, the poor is in reference not in finances, but poverty born of a shortage of ideas. This does not mean that we possess all the ideas in the world. It means we are open to find new ideas, from the books we read, from our friends and or from the seminars we attend. Somebody once said, "You are who you are because of the books you read and the people you associate with."

Trust the Process

Handstand is one of the poses that I enjoy doing in my practice, and it makes me feel good. It gives me a good indication of where I am in my practice and is a good measure of the balance between strength and flexibility. It is one pose that can be done without utilizing much space, especially if you are fairly good at it. However, it demands attention and persistent practice. You need to be able to feel your body from head to toe. Your foundation is your hands on the ground, and you depend on it all the way to your feet in the air.

To learn how to do a handstand is a process; the training has to be very specific and gradual. First, you must build your upper-body strength so that your wrists get used to holding your weight upside down. You need strong upper-arm muscles to withstand pressure and hold your weight together. Strong core muscles are needed to support the back and hold it in place. Lean and firm thigh muscles squeeze in toward the center and create one unified body. The same applies to your calf muscles, your feet and your ankles press together, all the way to your toes. All of this takes time to build up to. As I mentioned, it is a process. Working towards a handstand demands a certain way of working out—a formula that, when followed effectively, will lead you to your goal. How fast this happens depends on your physical shape and your background. I have chosen to use this analogy because it is the same with life, and how it worked out for me. As an acrobat and as a yogi, it took me time to achieve a handstand. It has taken even more time, and it still does, to maintain my handstand. And guess what? Fifteen years down the line there are some things that I am still working on.

Working on ourselves is a learning process that has no end. If I may borrow from WE, one of the core values is, "we are always learning." Working on ourselves demands that we are constantly checking to see how we are doing and how we can make an improvement in any given area of life. It is natural for us as human beings to check out from time to time, and that is why we have to keep bringing ourselves back to what really matters. Asking the right questions about ourselves and our situations, keeps us advancing in a process that has no end. We should not let ourselves settle, because if we do, then life automatically ceases for us. Growth demands that change. For change to happen, something has to give. Change is inevitable and constant, one way or another it is bound to happen and there is nothing you or I can do about it.

Our goal is to make sure that change happens in our favor. We have to stay in touch with who we are and constantly work on ourselves to bring the necessary changes and improve ourselves daily. Sometimes the process is not what we envisioned nor is it something that we would want. Sometimes it takes more time than we anticipated. When things get almost unbearable, we need to take a step back and breathe. Sometimes it is okay to trust in the process and keep at it at all costs until that which we want comes to be. It is darker towards dawn. When you start feeling that you cannot hold the pose anymore, that is when the pose starts working for you and that is when yoga happens. Maintain equanimity, especially in the storms. This is how the process works. It is being and learning how to be comfortable with the uncomfortable.

Consider that your growth will lie beyond your comfort zone. It is right at your edges. When holding a handstand or working on a downward-facing dog, you might feel some pins and needles in your upper arms and shoulders. This is just part of the journey and process; do not freak out. There is nothing wrong with how you are feeling or with you. You are not weak; it is just the way it feels and the language of the muscles. Listen with no judgment or favor. It is possible to move beyond it if you keep at it.

This morning I am working on handstand claps. This is a very new exercise for me. The first time I tried it I could hardly go beyond twenty-seven on a count. However, I have figured out a way that may help me get there. I have designed a work-out program to help me work effectively on getting the handstand claps for a challenge from a friend of mine who happens to believe that I can do it. The plan is to do a set of exercises every day for the next two weeks and see how effective it is, and then decide if I need to adjust my program or do something else altogether. This will involve holding forearm planks, v-ups, handstand kick-ups, and handstand holds for up to one minute or more. I figure if I could hold a handstand for more than a minute then I can easily do claps too.

This is the process so far and my belief is, if I follow it to the letter, then I will have a good shot at succeeding at my challenge. I need to trust the process and not expend anything less than the input of energy, time and concentration needed to see it through.

The Modern Warrior

The spirit of a warrior transcends the trials and tribulations of life as we see it or as it occurs to us. The warrior spirit chooses and tries not to operate from default. The warrior spirit makes a path where there is no path and is not afraid of being wrong. As a warrior, you learn to accept your downfalls and your victories with the same enthusiasm. As a warrior, you learn to accept others for who they are, to motivate them to use their strengths for the benefit of all. The warrior chooses positive, enabling, progressive thoughts that are empowering.

Let us look at the Maasai warriors and the lives they led before lion hunting was rendered illegal in Kenya. They hunted lions as a hobby, and as a show of manhood and bravery. They did this for such a long time that the number of lions dwindled over the years. Poaching and illegal hunting made the situation worse. The government intervened with a severe warning and imposed a penalty. It also offered an incentive for warriors who were interested in preserving and protecting Kenya's wildlife. The Maasai would give up part of their land for conservation and be paid a fee dependent on how much land was donated. Wild animals were then able to roam across the warriors' land—a sort of union between wild and domesticated animals, grazing side by side. Maasai cattle and sheep could be seen grazing together with wildebeests, zebras, gazelles, giraffes and many others. Thus, the Kenyan government was able to enroll the warriors' help in preserving the wild. Through this initiative, the Maasai warriors were able to understand how the killing of lions affected their economy. As Tim Cork says, "When people understand the 'why,' they understand the purpose, which always comes from the inside."

This example also suggests the kind of warrior we need to be in our modern societies. We need to be warriors that recognize, and move away from, small, negative talk—the internal voices that tell us that we cannot do this or that. We must work to suppress these invisible, self-trapping voices that hinder us from accessing the true power of who we are as a people and as a generation. We must move from a "me" to a "we" kind of warrior. We must recognize that empowering others is more powerful and sustainable than doing something alone in the hopes of attaining an individual win. If you want to go fast, do it alone; but if you want to go far, do it together with a lot of people on your side. The modern warrior realizes the longevity in doing things with others, as no man can exist on his own. "No man is an island," someone once said, and I couldn't agree more. As a person, you are capable of achieving a lot, but as a community, you can do much more than you might ever anticipate or perceive as possible.

If you allow me, I will take you back to how the Maasai warriors conducted their lion hunts. Hunts were carried out during a very specific time in a Maasai warriors' life, during their initiation into adulthood. Boys would go to the jungle in large groups "to become warriors." After spending months training, perfecting their hunting skills and learning the ways of the Maasai, they would be considered ready for a lion hunt that would mark the end of their training and graduation into a warrior. They would come dressed in their beautiful warrior gear made of cowhides; loin clothes that essentially looks like miniskirts, topless, apart from the beautifully made Maasai beaded chains running diagonally across their chests. Their entire bodies would be painted in red ochre. If you met one of them, they might scare the hell out of you. As a group, they surely had this effect on even the mightiest of lions. A small bell is strapped just above the knee and is kept wrapped under a piece of cloth until a male lion is spotted. Yes, a male lion. Now you understand why the lion population dwindled at such an alarming rate. After one or two Maasai spotted a lion, they would release their bells to alert the rest of the group to make a circle trap. They would then begin to lure the lion to the center of the circle of warriors. Slowly, they inched forward to a distance close enough to increase chances of success in the first throw, and without taking too much risk. Whoever threw the first spear that hit and injured the lion would be regarded as the lion killer, regardless of whether the throw was fatal or not. This warrior would be awarded the mane as the first prize. The second thrower would be awarded the tail and the rest of the group would be happy to be called warriors for just having participated in the hunt and eventual killing of the lion.

The Maasai warriors are known to be among the most fearsome African warriors. They know better than to approach or hunt lions as individuals. Instead, they operate in a group and a fearsome one at that. Human beings are like pack animals. We work better in groups. This is how we evolved many years ago. It's in our DNA. There is an African saying: "Togetherness is strength and division is a weakness." A true warrior has the energy and spirit of togetherness and shuns anything and anyone who does not recognize other people's contributions to matters of life.

Disrupting the Soil

Growing up with my grandma was both hard and interesting, as I got to learn so much from her. My gran was a loving, caring and tough lady who put up with a lot of life's hardships. She was a second wife, and much younger than her co-wife. There was a lot of bad blood between her and her co-wife, so much so that the two families needed to be separated. Fortunately, gran's children did well in school, but this only fueled the animosity between the two wives. My grandfather spent more time with her than he did with the other family. Trouble came when he passed on and left my gran with eleven children to look after. This was a huge challenge, but she never gave up. She was the strongest person I ever knew. She fought to make sure that the legacy of her husband continued by schooling all of her children. This was the only weapon she had against her co-wife, who after the death of their husband wanted to take all the land and divide it amongst her own children without considering the second family. Education became the only key to wealth that she could be sure of giving her sons and daughters.

As a seasoned farmer and small retail shop owner, my gran reminded me from time to time that unless you dig up the soil every season, nothing but weeds will grow. One day, I asked her why we had to do this when we could just make a small hole big enough to plant the seed. "The soil, after harvesting, stays undisturbed until the next planting season. In the course of this time, useless weeds take over. Without digging up the soil and creating a disturbance, the weeds will literally swallow and choke the new seed. The seed will never see the rays of the sun, and the farmer will go hungry. By disturbing the soil, you cut the life of weeds, at least for a while, loosen the soil and provide nutrients for the new seed, giving it a fair and fighting chance to grow."

As a grown-up, I have come to appreciate the deep lessons from my grandma. Sometimes, I get so absorbed in a certain way of doing things that I miss the impact it is creating. I fail to see how stuck I am. Digging up the soil is like disrupting the normal way of operating and being willing to learn new ways of dealing with adversity. It is like breaking up the routine and coming up with a new program.

In this age of information, we learn so much. Sometimes, it's important to unlearn so as to create space for new information. For every advancement, there must be some adjustment. Like my grandma said, "If we don't till the land, only useless weeds will continue to grow." Sometimes, if we don't change our way of thinking, we can remain trapped in our stories. History can both inform and trap us. We create stories from our history. Our stories are born of our interpretation of what happened in the past, which at times may be questionable, depending on our emotional state and maturity. And there is always the chance to create a new interpretation of the same situation in the present that will alter our stories. This is why it is not wise to rely on history alone to inform the choices made in the present. Both new and old information is vital in making a well-rounded, well-informed decision. Alone, the topsoil that produced last season's harvest is not nutritious enough to give us another bumper harvest. It must be worked; mixed up, loosened and disrupted in order for the new seed to germinate and produce another plentiful harvest the next year.

Highlights

If you are lucky, life is made up of endless days. As we live, we have different experiences each day, and we give each day a different title: good or bad. However, the days are just days, neither good nor bad, they just are, endless. Good or bad is the label we give them to suit or fit our description of how the day has occurred. Knowingly or unknowingly, the way we approach each day defines how the day will progress for us.

Highlights, in this context, are the things and moments that take your breath away; that capture your eye, captivate your imagination, hold you in a trance, and make you think and reflect on how life happens around us.

Some people have developed a culture of sharing days' highlights with those around them. This sharing not only allows people to see how different we all experience life, but it also shows that we all have varied perspectives of thought and thought processes. One's highlights might be completely different from that of others who are living similar life experiences. This explains how a day is just a day and is largely dependent on how you approach and live it. You might feel energetic or tired, happy or angry, excited or moody, and your day will simply roll to the tune of your thoughts and feelings.

So, your day is shaped from the inside out. Whatever thoughts and feelings you have will radiate from the inside and shape your outside world. It's the invisible creating the visible. And fundamentally, this is how everything is created or formed on earth. Your thoughts and feelings guide your approach to life and how you live it. As I said before, 10 percent is what happens to you in life and 90 percent is how you react to it—aka, your attitude. Your attitude is largely informed by your thoughts and feelings.

By sharing highlights at the end of each day, I acknowledge the good things that happened to me. By sharing out loud in a group or even to yourself, you are thinking about a moment or subject that you appreciate and want more of. The more we think about it, the more of it we attract in our life. The law of attraction says that we attract that which we think about most. What you focus on expands and grows, and so the highlights become another chance to focus on that which we want in life. When you voice your thoughts, it is like sending a signal to the universe that is interpreted and reciprocated in the same proportion as the amount of thought and feeling put into it.

Taking time to think about the things we like and appreciate in life is important in building the kind of life we want for ourselves and for others around us. Acknowledge people and their contribution to your life at the end of every day. Let them know that you appreciate them for who they are and for what they stand for as individuals. This way you will continually attract and keep people who are on the same wavelength as you, people who support what you stand for and who you are.

Life is like a spiral: that which you send out comes back in the same measure. This builds consciousness in how we operate from day-to-day. A conscious man creates a conscious life and a conscious environment where everything and everyone is supportive of one another. This is one's Utopia. By appreciating that which is available to us, we cultivate a sense of gratitude. With an attitude of gratitude every day—our highlights—we attract that which makes us happy and keeps us connected. The world would be a much better place if we all lived like this.

Relationships

Life is about relationships, and people are generally relational beings. You start by relating to yourself, and then to someone, something or someplace. The relationship that you have had with people has led to where you are in life. It's the dots coming together to form a curve of your life path. Sometimes, we don't stop long enough to see or appreciate the dots or milestones; the changes on our path as we move forward. When you take time to connect, see and appreciate these things, only then can you adequately say that you are having a close and good relationship with yourself.

I entered the field of art from a unique angle; an angle that had very little flexibility in terms of creativity. In fact, anything with a military influence in Kenya had very little room for art, apart from martial arts and few sports. An order or command has no two ways. An order does not have opinions, and it is not questionable.

Back when the team decided to train hard in acrobatics, I took the responsibility of pushing us into a high level of fitness and achievement in our field. My way of relating to myself was influenced by the strict discipline under the rule of command. I was the sergeant major, this time self-appointed. We had to succeed. Our cash was short and often we could not see how it would last as long as needed. We needed to make the most out of the time we had, and to come up with a salable product. I rode everybody so hard that they wished the ground would swallow me. I was good at listening to others, making suggestions and helping with decision making to create and form new human pyramids, as we called them. My job was to implement new workout programs, and I did my job well. I would make us repeat and repeat until we got it just right, or close enough. The next day, I demanded the same energy and dedication. I was a badass; I was on fire, No excuses. Everybody had to do their bit and no less. This is how we managed to do well and in record time. However, in this very space of time, I made enemies in my group.

In acrobatics, we cherish the uniqueness of every member. All of us in the group hold different positions and we need each other to execute the final performance. Everybody is different and that is the beauty of this act. I just didn't link that concept to how I dealt with my friends. This logic escaped me for the longest time. I did not figure out that our contribution was also based on our differences and uniqueness. My approach should have been more inclusive and accommodating.

My relationship with myself was unharmonious as well. I strongly believed in pushing my limits. I did not take the time to understand how this impacted the rest of the team. I was not in touch with myself enough to understand their feelings because I did not take the time to understand my own. My thoughts might have been well-intentioned, but the truth is that not all of us are built the same. We all represent our own uniqueness. I was hard on the others, and twice as hard on myself. I would hardly laugh at simple jokes. It was like I was uncomfortable smiling or laughing out loud. To me, smiling was an indication of being too relaxed or weak. I was constantly competing against myself. My comfort zone was being quiet and alone, even in the group. As a self-labeled disciplinarian, this was my norm, and it left little room for jokes. Truth is, I was intense, maybe too intense. My friends saw this, and I blocked them from coming too close because I feared I would lose my edge. Everything was working except that I was pushing my friends away. This weakened their morale and brought tension among the members, which is a very serious thing in our line of work as acrobats.

In African acrobatics, we rely on each other a lot. You cannot build a human pyramid alone. If you did, you'd have to come up with a new name for it. Not working together was not an option. Good morale means a lot in this context. Otherwise, somebody could cause a fatal accident. Negative energy multiples the chances of risk.

In a good talk with one of my friends in the group, he told me to ease off a little; to be more understanding and not pin people down so much when they do wrong or do less by my standards. I was good at pinning people in a corner, and I set high standards. I was harsh and unforgiving, a typical military attitude. It is different when you are the lead in a training program, but as a participant, this can be overwhelming. It is then that I started seeing the patterns and how they affected relationships with myself and with my friends. I wanted so much to relate to them all, but I thought that would compromise our mission. This relationship that I had with myself, largely informed by my past experiences, negatively impacted how I related to my friends.

Sometimes it is okay to stop and pause. This will give you a chance to catch your breath and find the middle path. When you take a pause, it's an application of the serenity prayer. There are things that we cannot change, and it takes courage to accept that. Sometimes we need to pause to find the energy to move on. The pause can help us find the center and the middle path to wisdom to know the difference.

Nothing to change, nothing to hide, everything to lean into. Embrace and enjoy the good, the ugly, the uncomfortable, the tedious, the funny, sad, and heartbreaking.

Learning how to relate to myself better is a continuous process and it gives me access to my own feelings. Now I understand that people get tired, and it does not mean they don't want to do something or that they are weak. They are just tired, and that should be okay. I understand why they felt the way they did.

Being in harmony with yourself is having a close relationship with yourself. It's being in touch with your emotions and choosing to operate from the present moment. This state of being creates good vibes around you, and as a result, good things and people are generally attracted to you. Relationships start from where we stand, yourself. How we relate to ourselves informs how we relate to others around us.

Building and maintaining good relationships bring you a step closer to your goals, and the direction that you want to go in life. It keeps the peace and avoids trivialities that will thwart and drag you down. Love yourself and it is bound to spill to others.

Packing

Eliminating extra weight is important when we want to fly. The extra weight pulls us down and reduces our speed. It also determines how far we can go and how much energy is spent on getting to our destination. Extra weight takes up a lot of space and does not allow much room for anything new that is acquired along the way.

The general rule of packing is: Pack half the things you think you'll need for your journey. This is easier said than done, for sure. I have always struggled with packing less than what I think I will need on my journey. However, there have been a couple of times when I have been able to pack just enough of what I'll actually need. On these occasions, I felt light, I worried less about losing my luggage. I had confidence I knew where everything was, this gave me so much peace. Most of the time, though, this has been difficult to do, and I've found myself with way more than I needed for my trip. This leaves me with a bad taste in my mouth as I know I can do much better. So, now there is no space for souvenirs, and as you know, in most cases when you travel you bring things home.

I remember one time when I traveled abroad, and I planned to buy little or nothing at all. For this reason, I decided that I needed to pack as many clothes as possible so that I wouldn't have to buy any extra. Man, have I ever been wrong! I realized very quickly into my trip that I had carried way more than I needed and that I had no space for anything else. And of course, I did make some purchases here and there. I ended up having to get an extra bag for the additional things that I bought: gifts for my children which I could not leave behind.

There is a theory that the way you do anything is the way you do everything. This scares me a little when I think about the things that I know I don't handle very well, and yet gives me confidence in things that I know I do well. Creating a balance; now this is an art. At the airport, I had excess weight and I was forced to either pay for the additional pounds or leave the extra weight behind. This happened a couple of times during my travels, and so maybe you can see why this had such an effect on me and why I choose to talk about it.

In real life, sometimes we have a lot of expectations for ourselves or for others. These demands can take away from the present moment and affect our ability to listen, be with others, and experience the situation as it is. The expectations that sit in the background come by default, most likely influenced by history or standards that you have unconsciously set for the situation. This means that you are missing out on the present moment experiences, and your contributions will be limited. I call this expectations overload. When you have expectations or extra unwanted weight, it puts you in a judgmental state. Being judgmental is like being biased, you only listen from one dimension, nothing good comes out of it. Drop your expectations and listen generously without creating and forming solutions as you listen. Drop the extra baggage so that you are light enough to fly with and be with the moment. See the situation as it is and not your misconceptions and your opinions of what you think it should be.

When we venture into unfamiliar grounds, which happens a lot, we tend to pack a lot. Among the things we pack is fear, particularly fear of the unknown. Everybody is afraid of something, especially what we don't know. It is hard to get rid of fear, but we must not overthink it. Fear is only bad when it stops us from doing and becoming the people we want to be. We can see fear as unwanted baggage, and yet it plays an important role. Fear that informs your choice with care is good. Fear that stops you from trying new things and taking risks that will open new doors is an extra weight that needs to be dropped.

First impressions are very important. A wrong impression can ruin your reputation and cost you an opportunity. The opposite of that is being trapped in the bubble of the concern of looking good. This will result in inauthenticity. If your goal is to look good, then you lose the authenticity of involvement. This clouds your mind and impairs your judgment. It's like having a spec on your eyes so that you do not see clearly. This concern is one other weight that needs to be set aside. You don't need this in your quest to advance yourself. When you pack, remember not to pack this concern of looking good. Leave out this extra weight.

Anxiety is another element that should be left behind. When you are anxious you cause panic and awaken fear that, among other things, takes you away from the real experience. We can definitely do without anxiety.

Overconfidence born of multiple wins and achievements can cause one to neglect the very things that can take him out or bring him up. Overconfidence breeds arrogance, clouding the mind, just like being overly concerned about the way we look. This is another weight not to take aboard.

Check your luggage to make sure that you've got half of what you think you'll need and put aside the unnecessary weight. Whether it is expectation, fear—fear that stops you from going for your heart's desire—the concern of looking good, anxiety, or overconfidence, remember what Baron Baptiste said: These are some of the "fixed perceptions that thwart and constrain us." Shed the extras and be ready to fly with the eagles, for you are an eagle!

The Konga

In the Maasai tribe and other Kalenjin tribes of Kenya, konga is a warriors' weapon. Sculptors make kongas from tree stumps found in the forest or bush. Under a tree, they chop the stump into big pieces at first to form the shape of the konga. Then, with a smaller ax, they start to chip away at the club. The sculptor then uses a smaller knife, a sharp broken piece of a bottle, and leaves from the sandpaper tree to finally bring out the beautiful konga.

The carving of a konga is similar to our lives, and how we seek to grow, become better people and achieve better results in what we do. It is a process of chipping away at the parts that don't serve us well, and forming the shape and size of the konga we want. It is a process that takes patience and consistent effort to see results. It's a process that cannot be rushed either, because if you do, you may end up chopping deeper than needed, and you'll have to start all over again on a new piece of wood. You must continue chipping, smoothing, and pausing from time to time to appreciate and acknowledge how your piece of work is progressing. Admire your work and your effort in changing its shape.

This process must continue until you expose the beauty that lies within the konga. Chip away at your habits and thoughts that are not supportive of your course. Move away from friends that hold you back and actions that are counterproductive to the progress you want. Continue to do this until you've exposed the gold—the konga—that is inherent in each and every one of us. And remember, "We are all standing in our own acres of diamonds, we have but to look."

Dig away, starting from where you stand.

When Life Shakes You

After all, is said and done, remember this statement I've repeated many times: History repeats itself. After all these years of turmoil and small wins here and there, I still find myself in vulnerable positions in life. It can be very scary and unforgiving, especially if you happen to come from where I have been. There have been drastic changes in the organization that I work for. Cost-cutting, they call it. I fell victim to the circumstances. My pay was severely reduced, and the effect was devastating. This, as you can imagine, was very heavy and harsh on my family. I had put all my eggs in one basket, so to speak, and now have lost most of them. I have the usual urban struggles of loans, school fees, and other bills to pay.

For the past two years, life was becoming normal, and I was getting used to managing my wages comfortably. Then this bombshell happened that triggered a memory from the past. For a span of days, I could not reconcile with the truth that this was happening. All I saw was my wife and kids on the street, languishing in poverty, just like I was during my youth. This thought scared me so much, I developed goosebumps every time I thought about it. My whole body would shake with pent up emotions that I'd held in for a long time. I pictured the hard and tough moments that I went through to get to where I was, and I couldn't believe I was so close to going back on the streets again. I took long walks, trying to wrap my mind around this and to think of a way out, but all I could see were my children's faces, innocent, unknowing. In a matter of days, I had been reduced to a pile of misery, and I hated putting myself in this compromising position. I hated everybody for being cheats; hated life for being unfair. I just wanted to scream out loud, or better yet, for the earth to open up and swallow me alive. This way I wouldn't have to explain where I disappeared to. Strange how things and events can scare you in this life!

Technically, I was still working, but there were significant changes in my wages. The amount I was left with was only sufficient to pay my monthly bills. You must then see that what was disturbing me was not the change itself, but rather what I made it mean. This, to me, was destabilizing, demeaning, disrespectful and unkind. How could anyone do this to me when I have given so much to my work? There has to be more than what meets the eye, I told myself. Somebody is against me and they are out to get me. They want to make me suffer or they just don't like me. I came up with so many theories to support and justify the results. Nothing seemed to make sense. I forgot the expression, "When it rains, it rains on everybody."

However, the facts are, it's business. There are tough times and some people will have to be laid off. Tough decisions are made, like the one that reduced my pay. My suffering is born of the stories I have told myself about this situation and what I have made it mean to me and my family. The sooner I notice this trend of thought, the sooner I will have the choice of starting a plan that will see things take a new turn or continue to suffer from my story. What is your story?

See, pain is inevitable, but suffering is a choice. From time to time we come across situations that are painful in life, and this is unavoidable. However, we continue to suffer because of the stories we tell ourselves about what happened. We have the choice to drop our stories and remain with the facts, which in real life are not that hard to comprehend. What stories do you tell yourself about what is happening or what has happened?

If there is one thing that yoga has taught me, it is that we perceive life through our five senses. Our sensations cause us to react in certain ways. We decide that something is bad or good depending on how we interpret it. One time we can decide something is good, and the next we decide it is not good. As a people, we are not consistent in our decisions.

Through conscious practice and learning, I have come to understand that these reactions bring about misery. To good sensations, I develop cravings, and with bad sensations, I develop aversions ,or hatred. I realized that I had generated a dislike, or even hatred, to a pay cut and what it means. This negativity made me suffer and become miserable. If I had had no attachment to my earnings and had surrendered to the law of the ever-changing phenomenon, I would have known that this like all other sensations, will pass, and therefore free me from my suffering. This would then give me space and time to concentrate on what's next without the interference of what's in the past.

The only way to be happy is to find ways to deal with these uncomfortable situations in life, informed by our sensations and recognizing our reactions. I am not saying that this is easy, but it is why I think yoga is a lifestyle, a journey, and a work in progress. It is about living in a conscious way that doesn't react to sensations. The old stock of aversions or cravings will keep coming up and disappearing. As we grow better in resisting to react to them, they become weaker, feebler and eventually get eradicated. This sets a path out of my self-created misery: observing the sensations that inform my feelings and emotions patiently, ardently and objectively, with the knowledge of the ever-changing phenomena that nothing lasts forever. With a perfect understanding of the universal law of impermanence, the situation is therefore defused from a mega-bomb into a non-substance, non-solid that is bound to change. With this in mind, suffering is taken out of the equation, or at least it lessens.

Yoga brings awareness of the mind and body; mind-consciousness, mastery, and purification of the mind so that one can build on the foundation of good moral values, which are universal.

Things are not any easier now that I do yoga and believe in the science behind it, but I have a better understanding of what is happening around me based on the experience and the truth within the framework of my body—reality is as it is, not as I want it; I exist from moment to moment, breath by breath. With this knowledge, it is easier to accept the things that I cannot change, to change the things I can, and have the wisdom to know the difference.

Today, I am working patiently, persistently, and diligently to develop wisdom in the art of living through the perfect understanding of the ever-changing phenomenon, the law of impermanence. I do this with underlying truth, attained not from the Bible or any Holy Koran, but within the framework of my own body. I seek liberation from the chaos and misery brought about by my own sensations.

I invite you to listen to your sensations and be aware of how they can lure you into a never-ending rollercoaster of emotions that keep you forever miserable. Getting out of this madness and helping others do the same so that we can all find happiness is my purpose, the push and the motivation behind all this.

Discover who you are and find your purpose. Find peace.

Acknowledgments

I dedicate this book to all the women in my life, beginning with my lovely wife and friend, Agnes Njeri Wanjiku, and my two beautiful daughters, Lauryn Chilande Cheloti and Elsie Wanjiku Cheloti. To my late grandma, Regina Nasike Wanyama, for taking care of me and making me the man I am today. My mom, Mary Khanjila Wanyama, for working so hard to educate all six of her children while juggling the challenges of a single mother. My aunt, the late Cate Simiyu, for taking care of me when I first came to the city and had no one else to run to. To my aunt Irene, such a darling friend.

My dear friends Kristen Bentley, with whom I have shared so much, and who offered immense guidance and encouragement on the writing of this book, and Amy Treichel Brand, who actually asked why I hadn't written something already. My lovely friend and soulmate Audrynne Mukami Ireri who helped with editing and made sure I wrote in English rather than translate from my mother tongue.

Biggest thank you to Cass Stillman and the Stillman family,

without whom this book would never have seen the light of day.

My uncle Bart Wanyama for being my father figure from when I was young and to all my other uncles. My teachers Baron Baptiste and Paige Elenson, the founder and director of the Africa Yoga Project. My mentor Suzie Newcome, founder of Namaspa Yoga Studio and Foundation in Oregon, USA.

Tim Cork, who played a major role in shaping this book as it is and for inspiring me with his words of wisdom.

Franco Lombardo, the one behind the inspiration and the push for writing this book. I will forever be indebted, my friend.

My friend and young brother, Isaac Mukwaya Vuyiya—together we have come quite a distance in our yoga journeys. My AYP friends, Walter Mugwe, Catherine Njete, and the hubby rasta Kiragu and sister Wanji, Nyakinyua, Yubra, Thairu, Basilio and Sadik. I have had immense support from all of you and the entire Kangemi crew, "the cultured."

And to my most valued friends, brothers in arms and my keepers, the entire Zamasimba crew members and pioneers, Job Ndirangu, Kariuki Kimani of Coro FM, Rasta Samson Njuguna, Jnr Mwangi, Mwai Wai, kijana mdogo Obach Madaga machachari, Michael Karanja Nganga, Mathu James Ben Waiyai and all the rest of the Kayole crew. And finally Mirema training grounds for creating such a support structure and contributing to my life in a way no one else has.

I salute you all, my friends, especially those that I have not mentioned. You mean the world to me.

Blessed love.

www.ingramcontent.com/pod-product-compliance
Lightning Source LLC
Chambersburg PA
CBHW020427010526
44118CB00010B/464